# The New Graduate Nurse's Survival Handbook:
## How to Avoid Being Labeled as "Scary"

**Jennifer Ensign Wilson**
**MSN, RN, CPN**
**Illustrated by Laura Hughes**

INFINITY
PUBLISHING

ISBN 978-0-7414-7020-1 Paperback
ISBN 978-0-7414-7021-8 eBook

Printed in the United States of America

Published March 2012

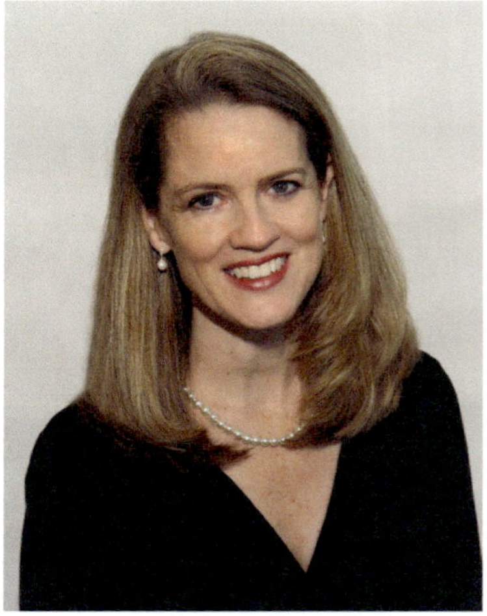

Jennifer Ensign Wilson
MSN, RN, CPN

INFINITY PUBLISHING
1094 New DeHaven Street, Suite 100
West Conshohocken, PA 19428-2713
Toll-free (877) BUY BOOK
Local Phone (610) 941-9999
Fax (610) 941-9959
Info@buybooksontheweb.com
www.buybooksontheweb.com

**Congratulations!** You survived nursing school and are about to embark on your nursing career. This book is intended to help you not only survive your new graduate experience, but to also get the most out of it as possible. Many of the common pitfalls of being a new graduate can be avoided by following the suggestions in this book. Share the book with your preceptor; it is sure to open up communication and generate some good discussion. Remember to keep a positive attitude and a sense of humor. I wish you the best of success in this exciting time of your nursing career!

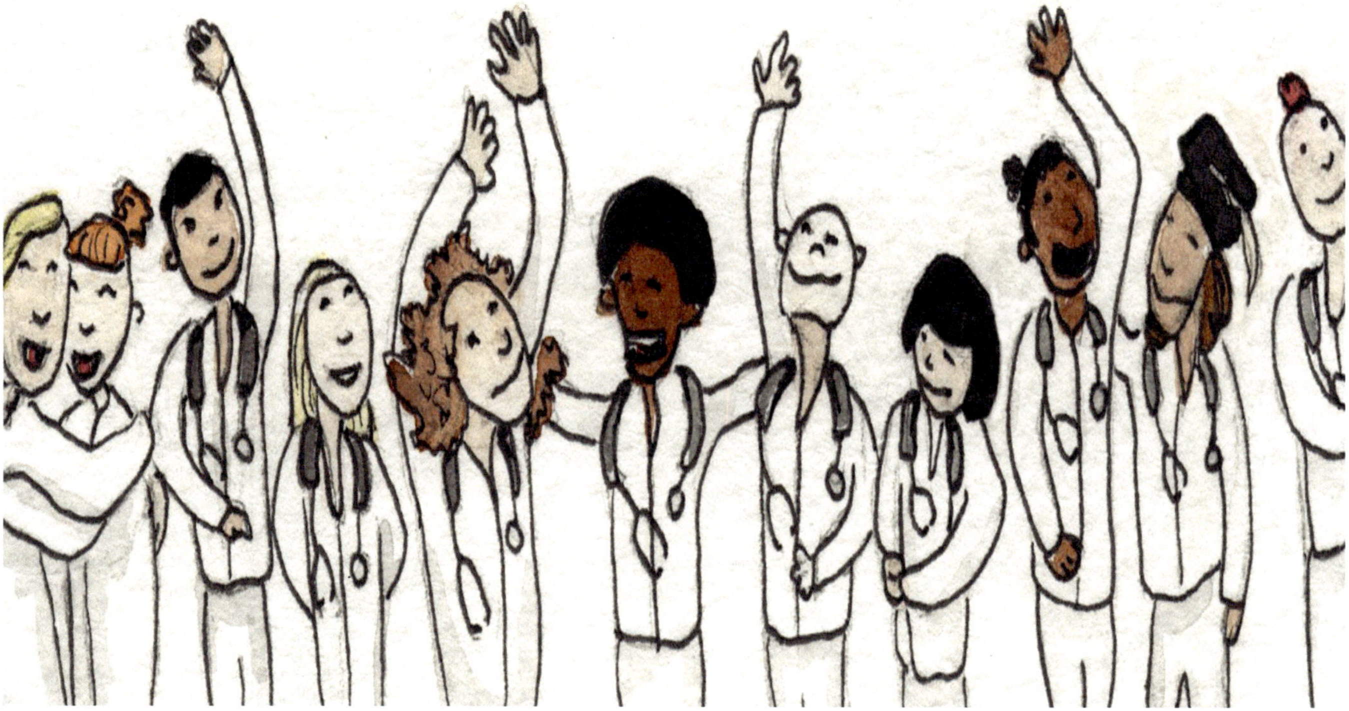

# BE HUMBLE AND TEACHABLE

Know that how you present yourself on the first day can affect the outcome of your new graduate experience. On your first day of orientation, tell your preceptor, "Assume I know nothing; teach me what I need to know to be successful on this unit." This does NOT mean "I know nothing" - it just shows you're teachable.There's nothing more annoying to some experienced nurses than a cocky new grad; it's an invitation to get chewed up and spit out.

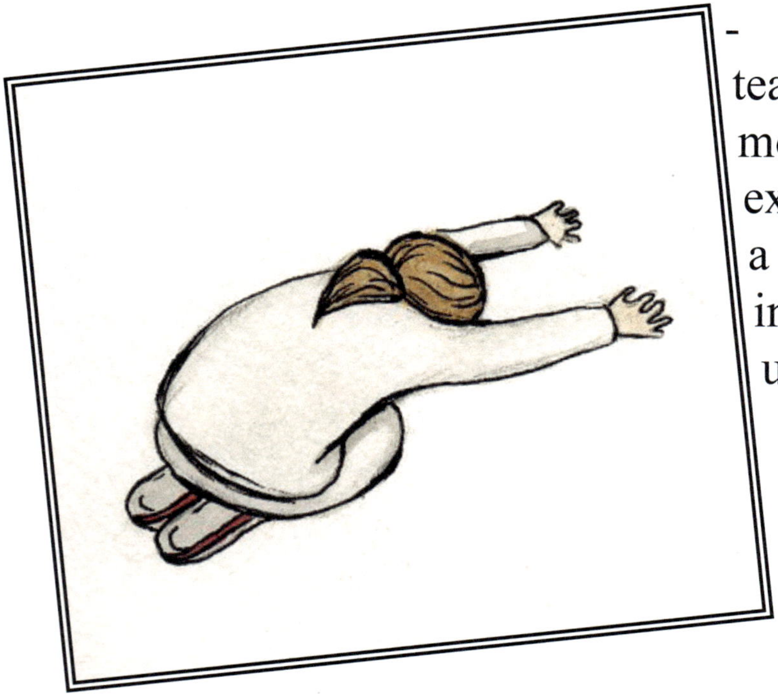

# TAKE ADVANTAGE

of the fact that you're a new graduate. People don't expect you to know everything - this is the time to soak up as much as you can. People will be much more willing to help you if you acknowledge that you have a lot to learn. Avoid saying "I know" a lot; it will cut off communication. Instead, nod and say, "okay."

Ride the wave.

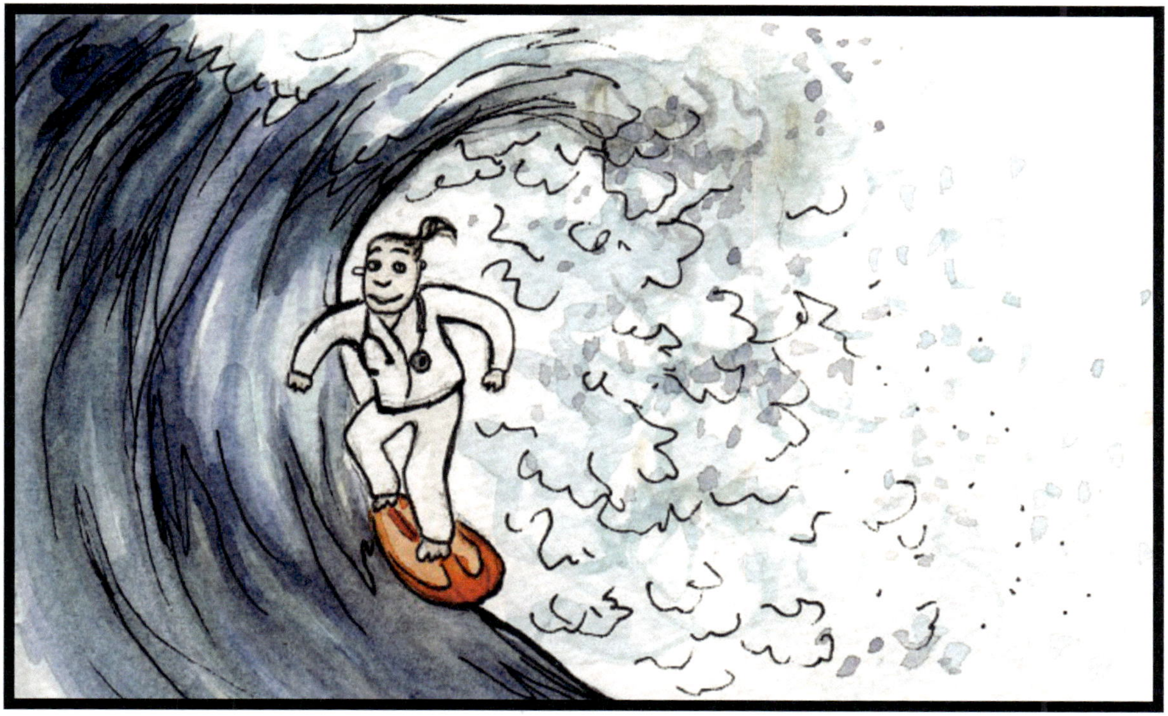

# THINK, THINK, THINK.

Constantly ask yourself "Why?" and "What will happen?" every time you are about to do something to, on, with or for a patient. If something does not make sense, stop and question it. There are some things that you simply cannot undo or take back once they're done. Never underestimate the consequences of your actions, or disregard when your "gut" tells you something.

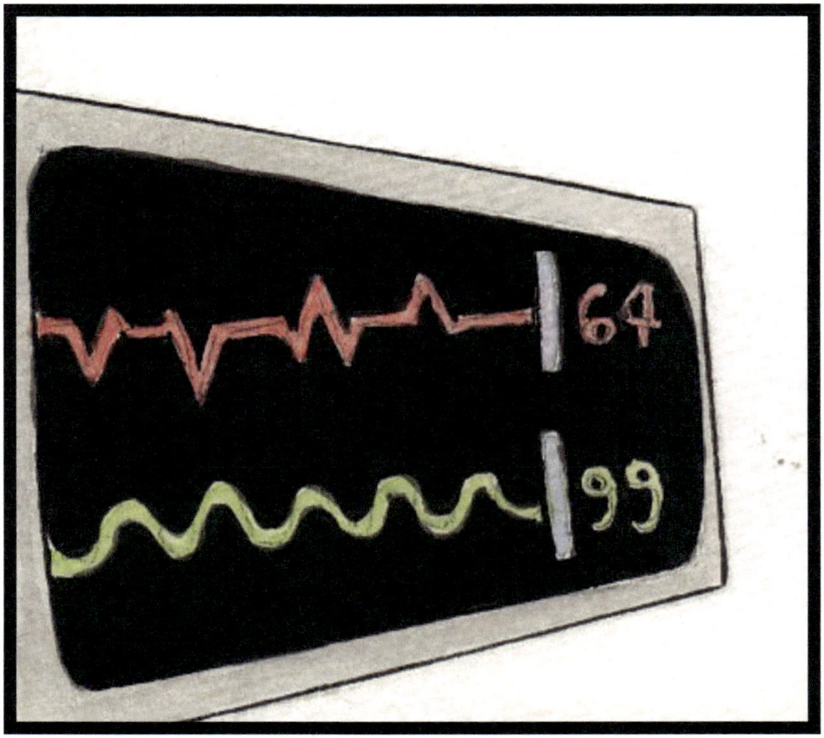

# ADMIT WHEN YOU MESS UP

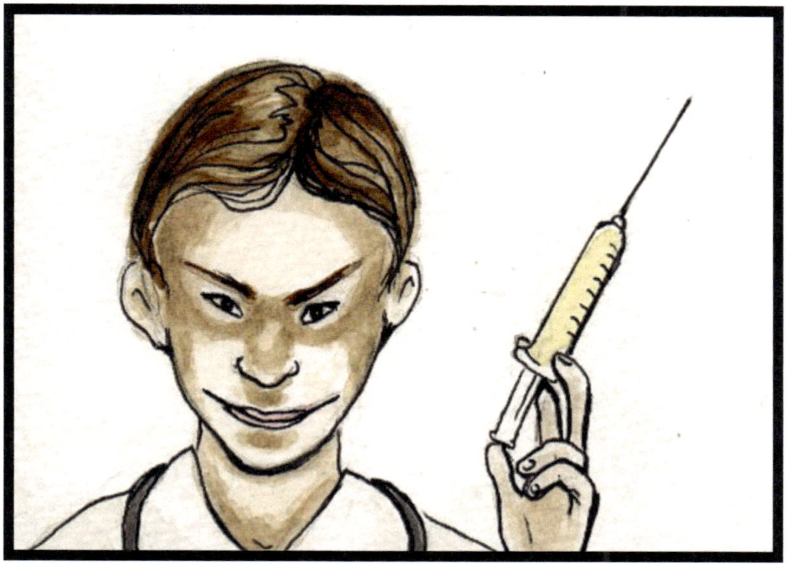

and tell others so that they will learn also. Go out of your way to tell your preceptor, charge nurse and manager if you make a mistake. They will trust you more if they hear about it from you than from others. If you try to hide or cover up something, you will be labeled as "scary."

# KNOWING WHAT YOU'RE DOING

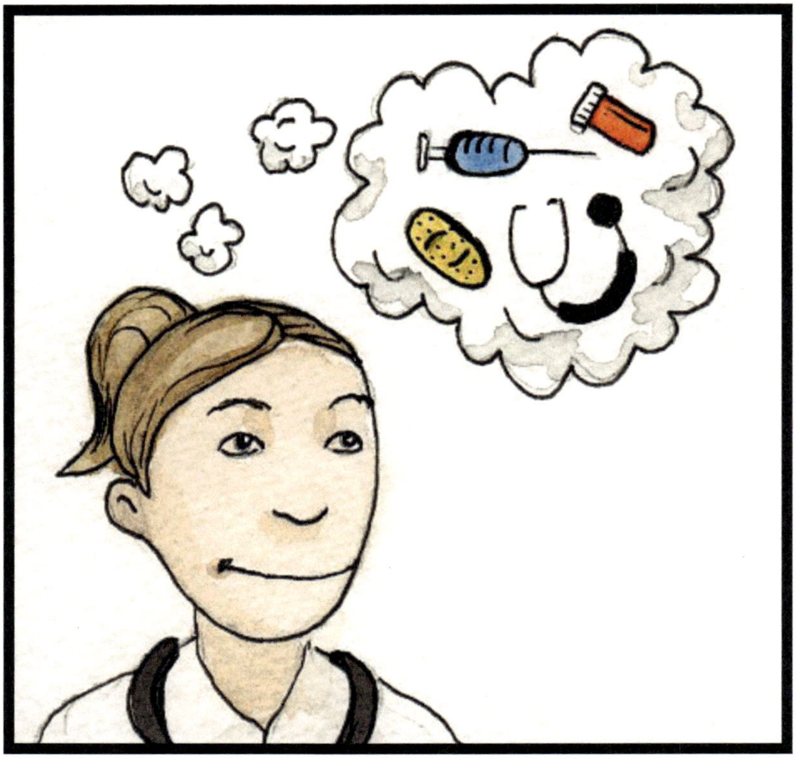

clinically is the first and most important step to being a fabulous nurse. Being kind, compassionate, empathetic and caring are really important, but they are not enough if you don't know what you're doing clinically. Know and practice within the boundaries of your license. Recognize when you need help, and don't be afraid to ask for it.

# REMIND YOURSELF EVERY DAY.

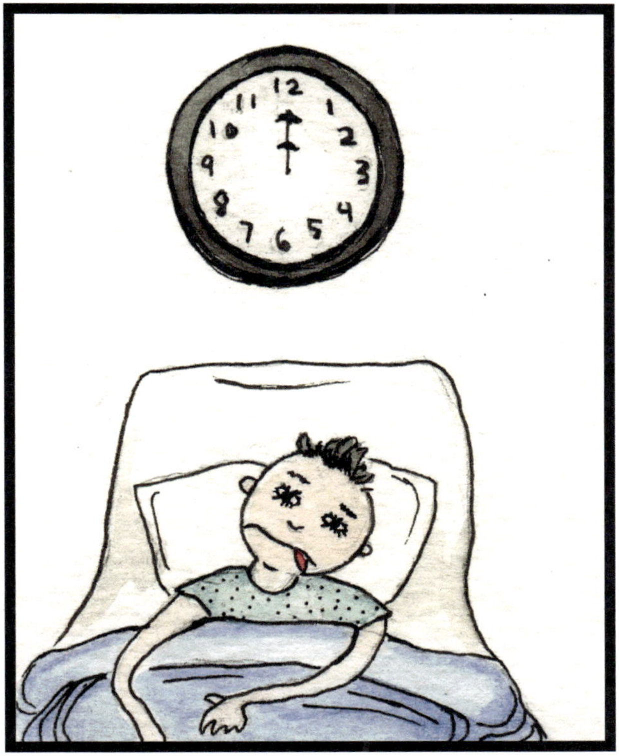


Remind yourself EVERY day that what we do as nurses MATTERS. And HOW we do it matters even more. How you look at your day changes everything. Approach your day as a 12-hour opportunity to make a measurable difference in your patients' lives. THEN DO IT. Wonderful things will come back to you in return.

# BE OPEN AND HONEST

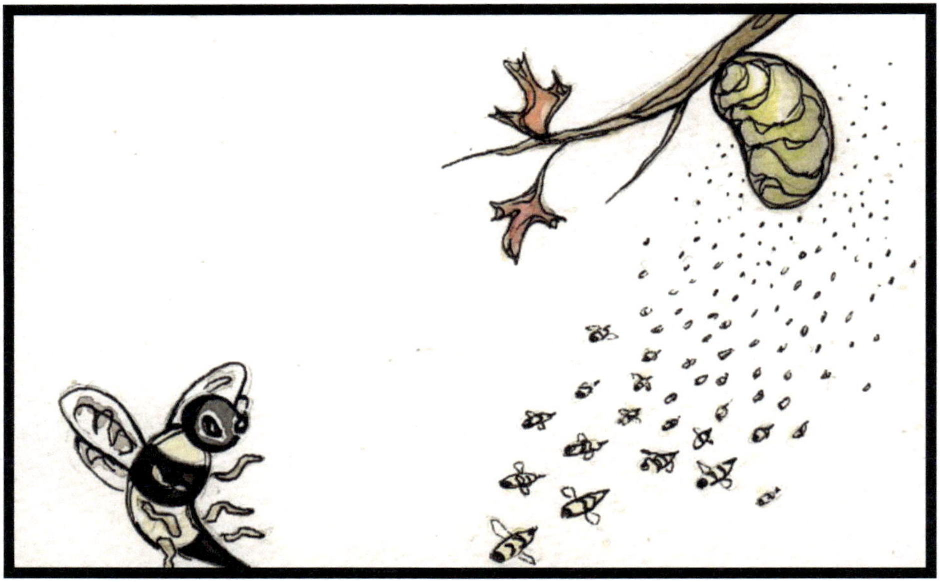

with your preceptor. DO NOT talk behind people's backs. If you have an issue with someone or how your orientation is going, follow the appropriate chain of command. If you badmouth a nurse, especially your preceptor, you run the risk of having a "swarm of bees" after you. Be a team player.

# BE PROFESSIONAL

at all times. Please show your patients that you care. Going the extra mile, rather than just doing your job, is what gives you that "nursing high," a jump in your step on the way home, and reminds you why you chose to be a nurse. It's the little things that will set you apart from the others. People really do notice.

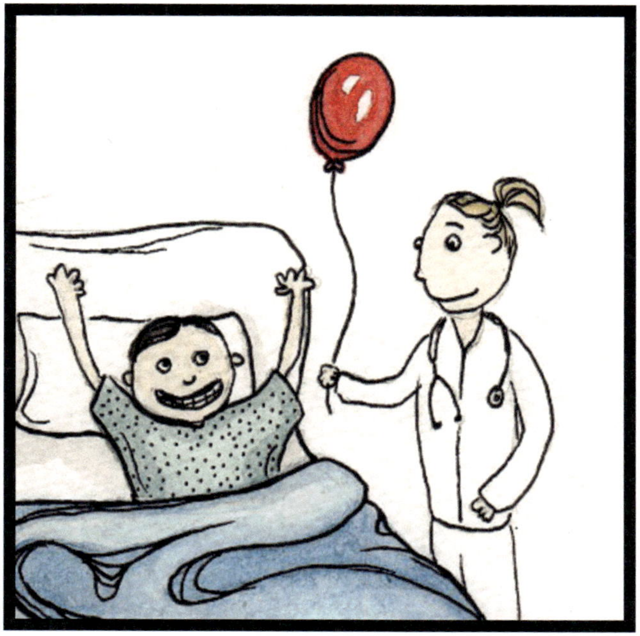

# ASK

if you are unsure about something. You will gain trust and respect faster if you show you are a thinker. Talk to physicians, nurse practitioners, respiratory therapists and pharmacists every day and ask them questions. The knowledge you will gain and the relationships you will form are invaluable. Also, stay in the room when physicians or nurse practitioners are talking to your patients - you will learn so much!

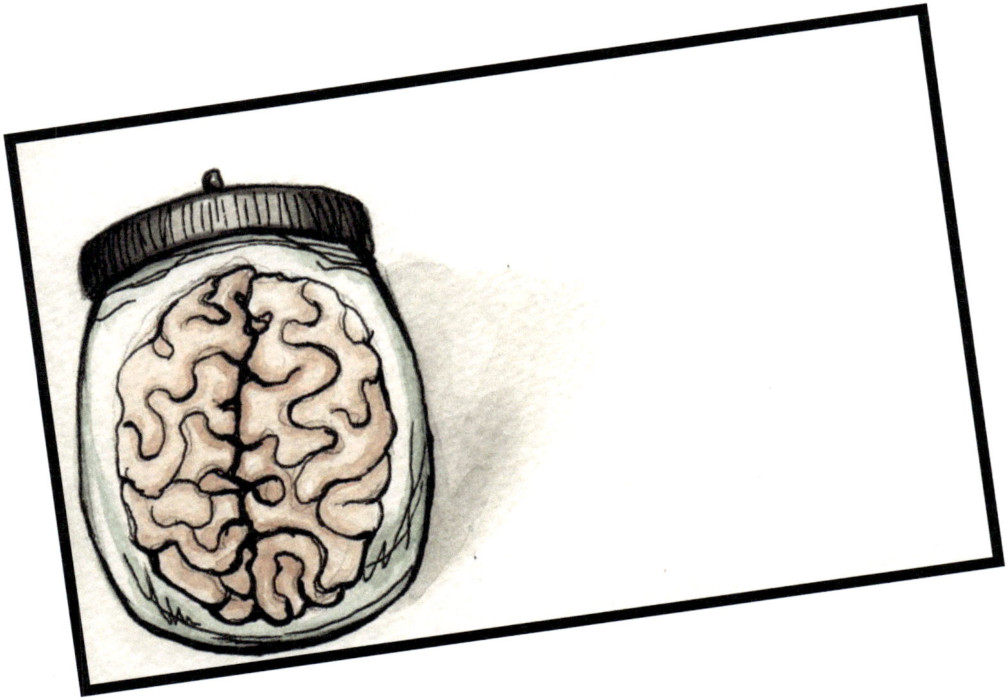

# MAKE SURE YOUR ASSESSMENTS ARE THOROUGH AND FREQUENT.

You're never really done with assessing, and before too long, you won't be able to look at patients <u>without</u> assessing them. Train your brain to take a "snapshot" picture when you assess to help you remember details. Be meticulous; check all your tubes going into and out of your patients from "bag to body" and know what's going on with them. Anything can happen!

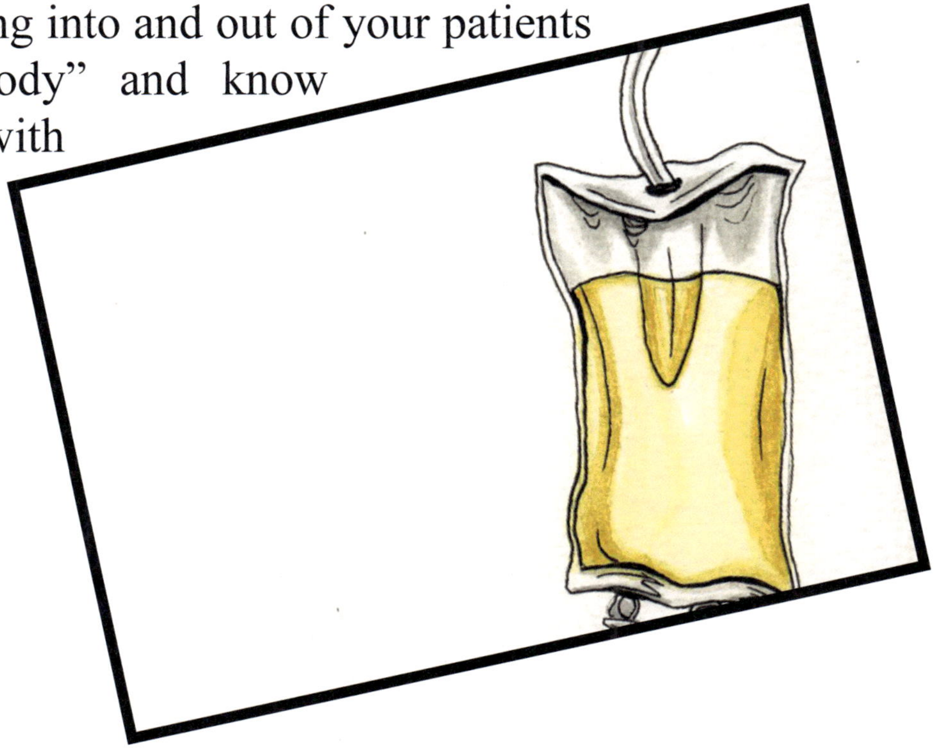

# BEFORE YOU BEGIN

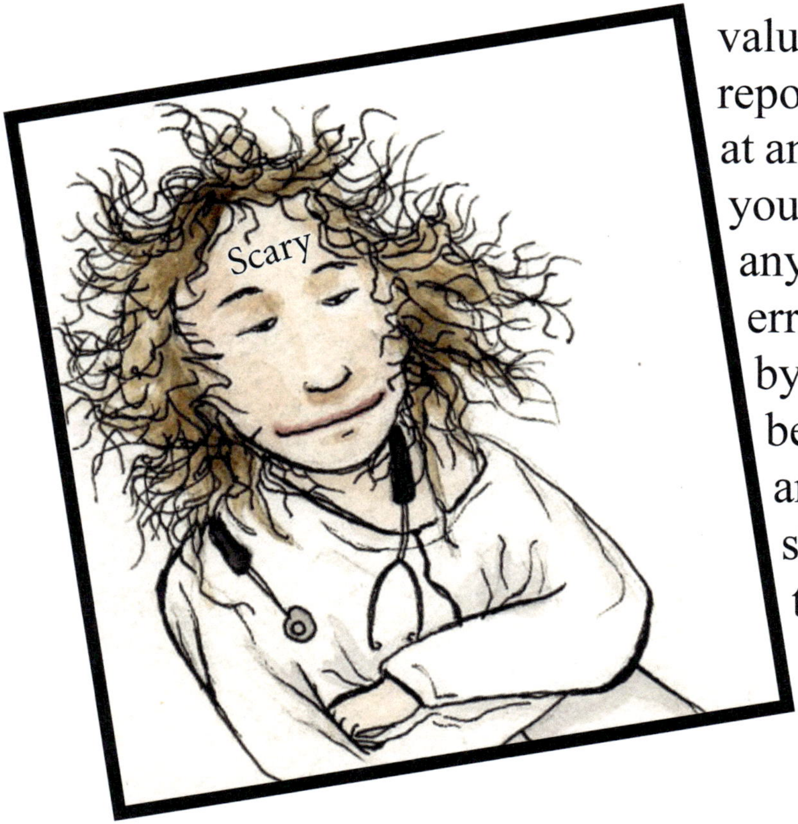


your shift and even touch your patients, look in their charts for recent orders and know their current lab values. Before you give report to the next shift, look at any orders written during your shift and pass on any pertinent info. Many errors can be avoided by doing this at the beginning, throughout, and at the end of your shift. Failure to do this can make you a "sloppy" nurse.

# ALWAYS TRY TO LOOK AT THINGS FROM THE PERSPECTIVE OF OTHERS.

This will help you key into what they need and how you can make a difference. Remember that **forethought** and **thoughtfulness** are the keys to making a difference. They are proactive, rather than reactive.

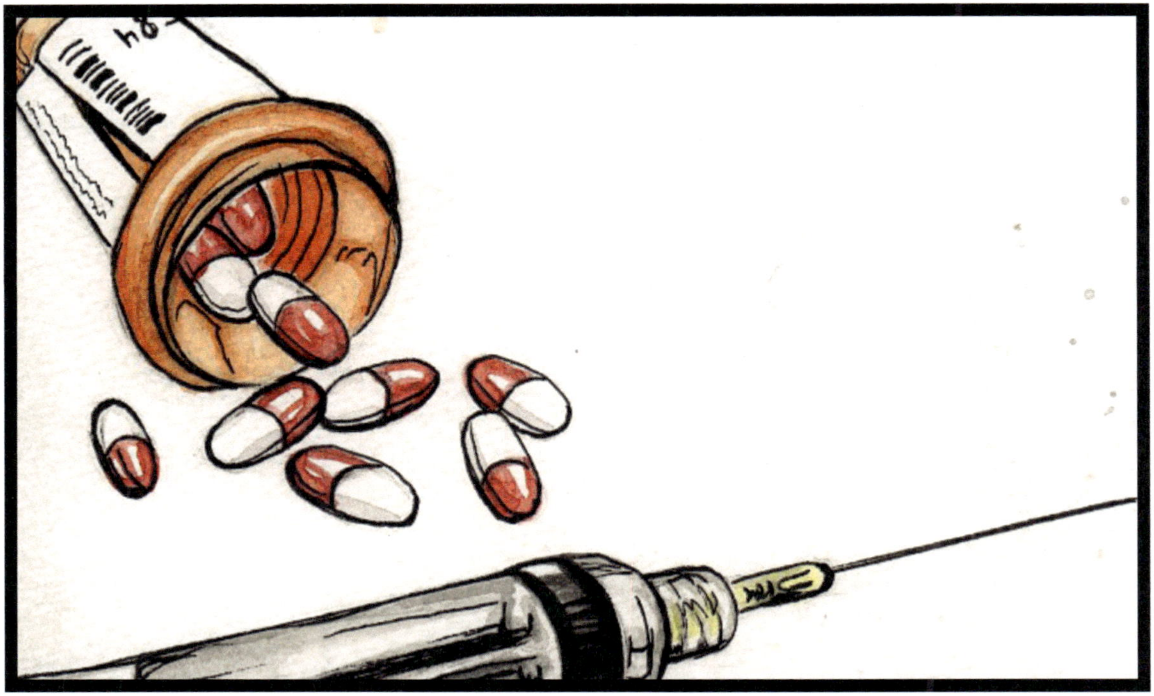

# DOUBLE AND TRIPLE CHECK YOUR MEDS.

You can never look at a medication too often or be too careful, regardless of how long you've been a nurse. If a nurse asks you to double check something for him or her, give it your undivided attention. If you can't, then tell him or her to find someone else to do it. There is a reason that certain meds need to be double checked and co-signed.

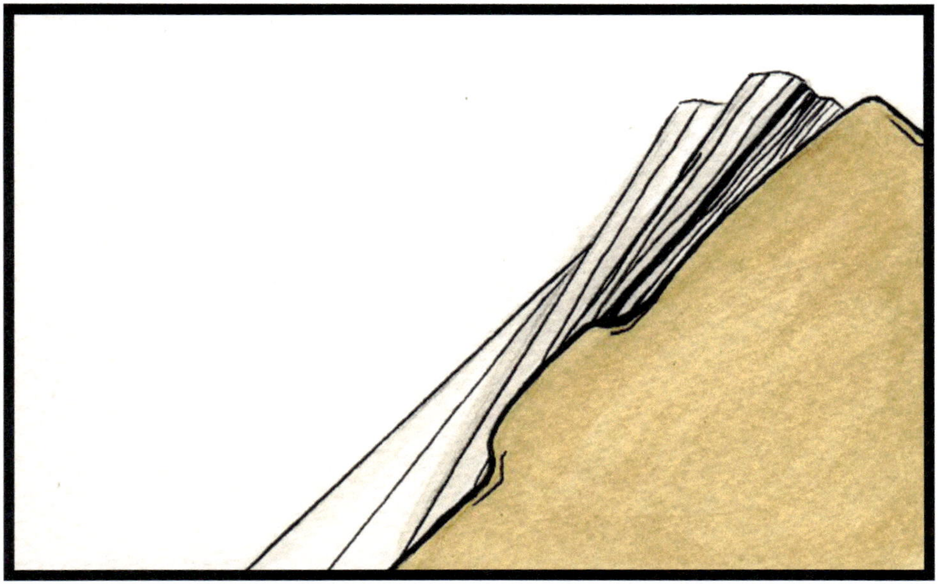

# WHEN YOU MAKE YOUR FIRST MED ERROR,

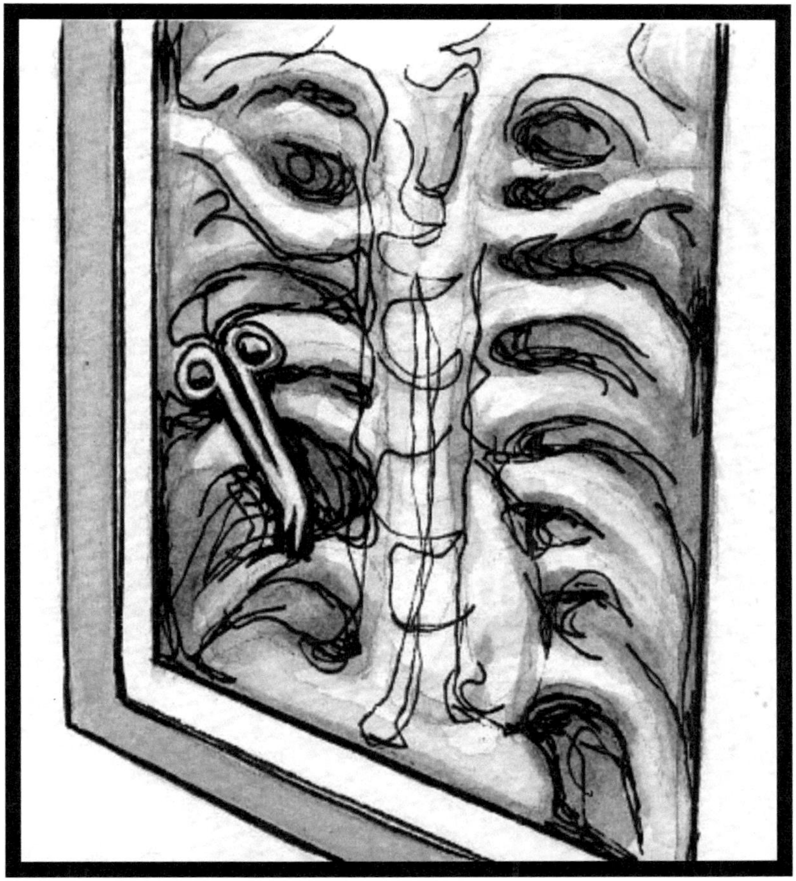

CARE, and act like you care, but try not to beat yourself up. You should be appropriately mortified, but still able to continue doing your job. If you act like it's no big deal, your preceptor might raise an eyebrow. Most importantly, take responsibility for your error and figure out how to keep it from happening again.

# EMBRACE YOUR MISTAKES AS INCIDENCES THAT MAKE YOU A BETTER NURSE.

Without question, my first med error made me a better nurse. Accept the fact that you will make mistakes, regardless of how hard you try not to. Learn from those mistakes and change your practice so that they don't happen again. Expect to encounter some challenging and difficult days as a new graduate. Those are often the days we grow the most, as painful as they can be at the time. Then return to work the next day a smarter and better nurse.

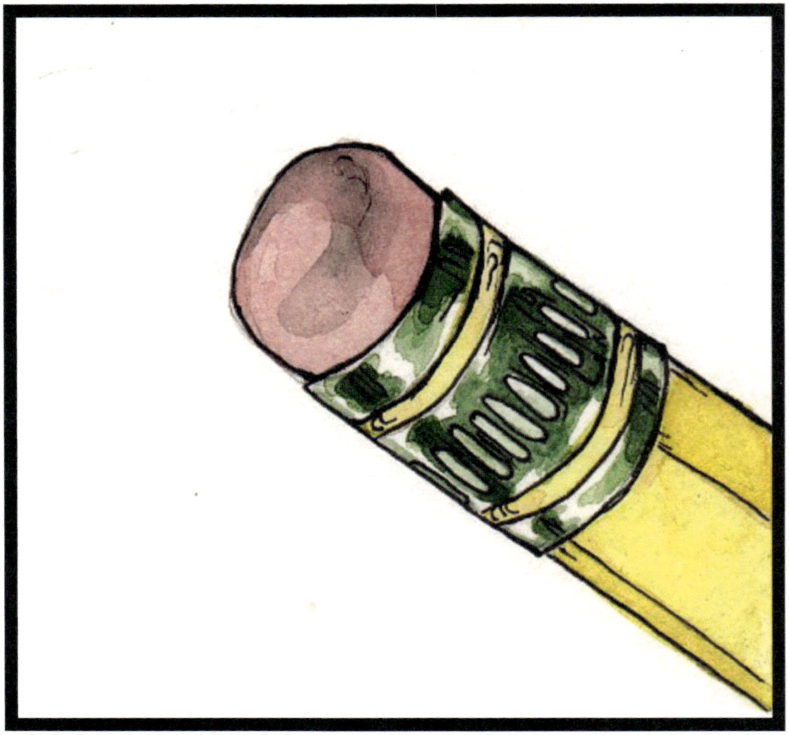

# DO THE RIGHT THING.

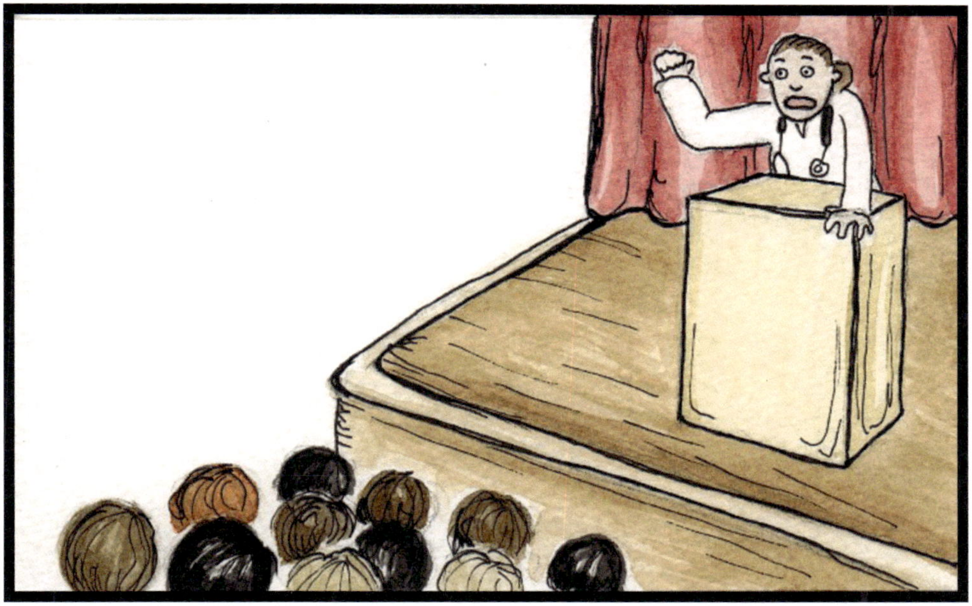

Advocate, advocate, advocate. If you were the patient, what would you want your nurse to do? If you know you are right, be diplomatic, but don't be afraid to stand up and fight for what's best for your patient. Be prepared to back up what you're saying with something in writing, like a policy or an article.

# MAKE A CONSCIOUS DECISION TO BE HAPPY.

The reality is that this can be a tough time of transition. Let's face it: nursing is a demanding profession, and the learning curve as a new graduate is huge. A positive attitude and <u>deciding</u> to be happy can be priceless. One of the keys to that is keeping the focus on your patients, rather than on yourself. You will be amazed at what comes back to you in return when you do.

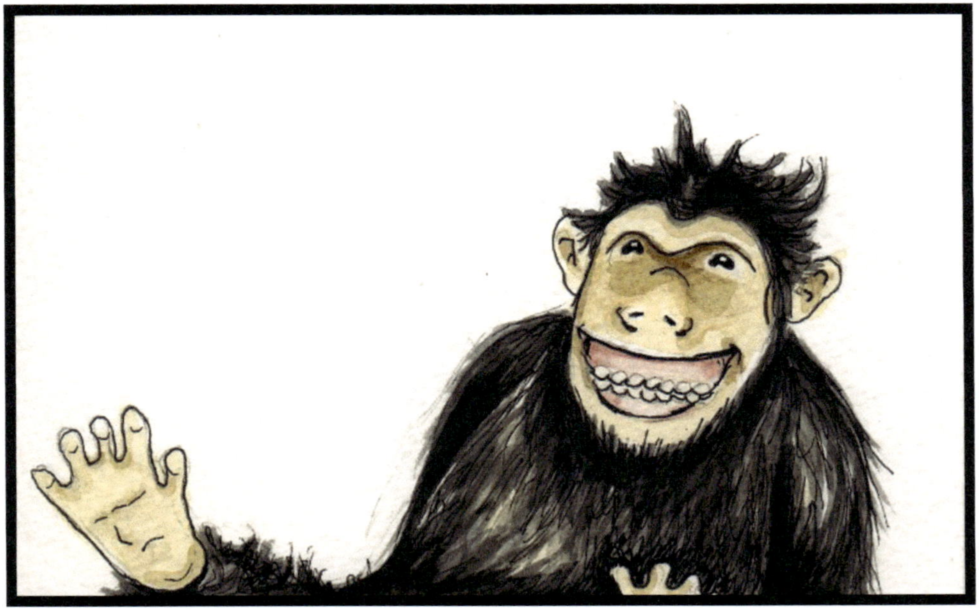

# LISTEN MORE THAN YOU TALK.

Resist the urge to to talk excessively about how you did things in school or at your last job. Try to look at things from the perspective of your preceptors, and thank them often for their patience, wisdom and knowledge. It takes a lot of energy to be a preceptor. Gratitude can go a long way, and will serve you well in this profession.

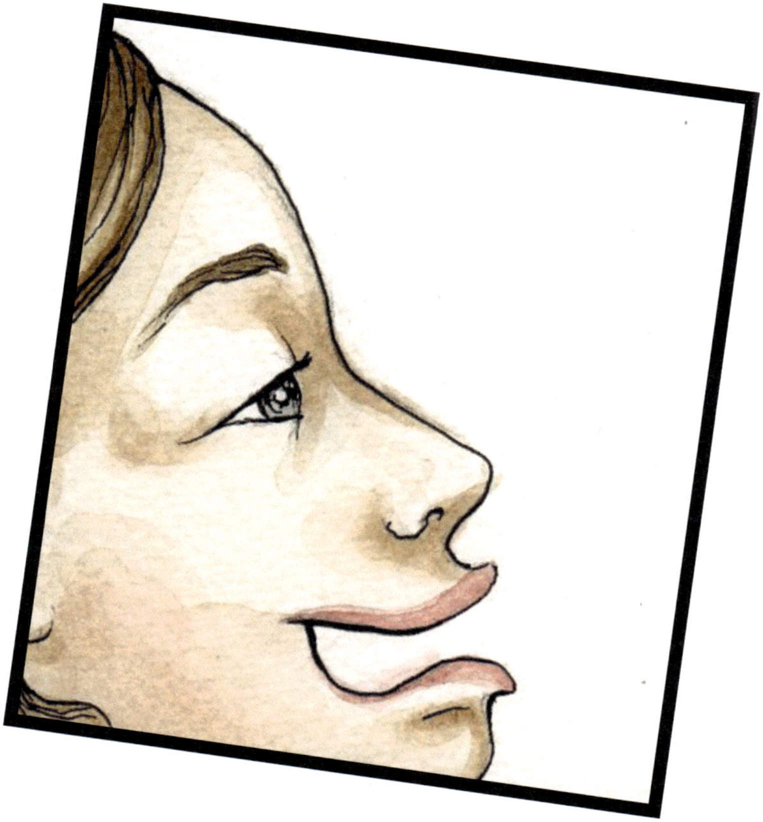

# SHOW PEOPLE THAT YOU WANT TO DO THINGS THE RIGHT WAY.

Whenever you are doing something for the first time, ask your preceptor to watch you do it. This shows confidence and will help the staff trust you. Understand that your preceptor's job is to ensure you are competent and meeting the expectations and standards on that unit. Your preceptor wants you to be successful. Realize that when you look good, your preceptor looks good. Once you and your preceptor agree you are competent to do something on your own, take the initiative and have the confidence to do it independently.

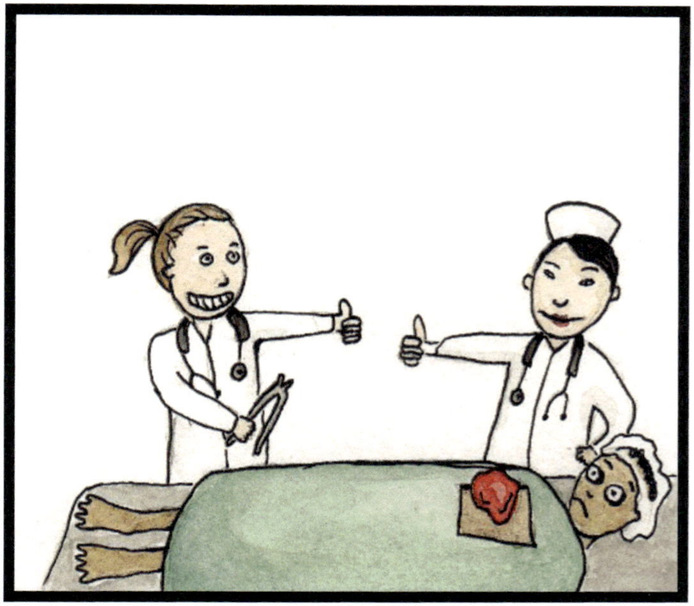

# INTEGRITY IS YOUR BEST FRIEND AND THE KEY TO BEING TRUSTED.

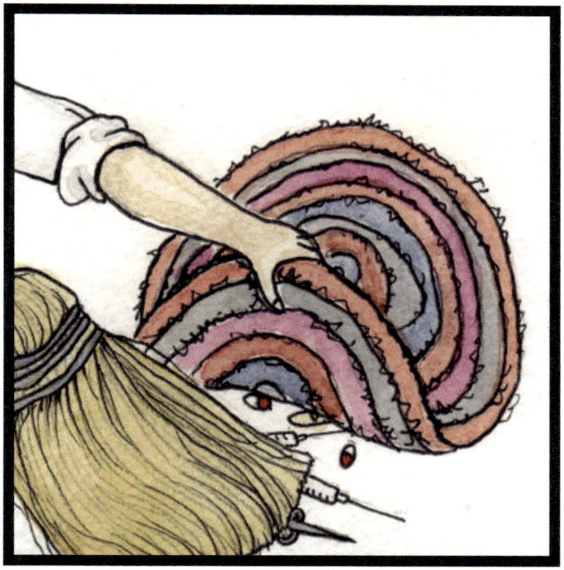

Model your practice after the exemplary nurses (they are usually the ones who are in their patients' rooms, rather than hanging out at the nurse's station). Pay attention to what makes them stand out and then magnify your own gifts and talents to be your own version of exemplary.

# DO WHAT YOU LOVE, LOVE WHAT YOU DO!

If you don't love your area after giving it your best effort for at least a year, try a new specialty; that's one of the beautiful things about nursing! If you are unhappy, do not bring others down with you. Keep life in perspective and remember what's important every day. Stay balanced and healthy, and fill your days off with good things.

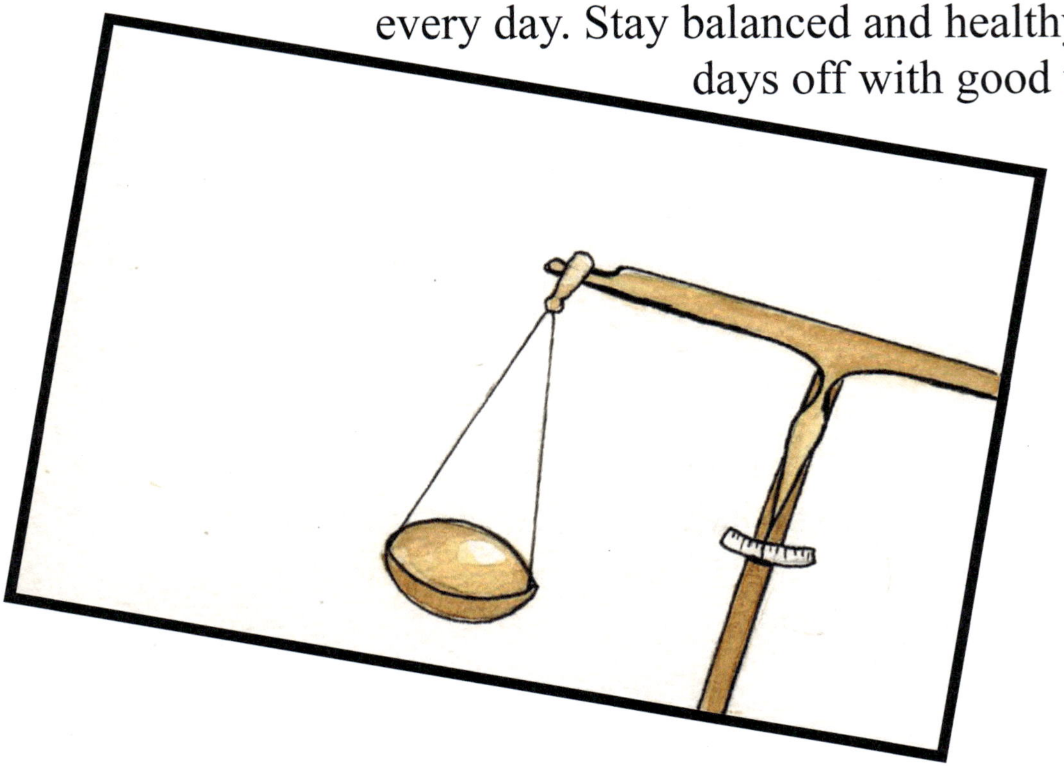

# ALWAYS REMEMBER WHAT IT FEELS LIKE

to be a nursing student and a new graduate. Treat those entering the profession behind you with kindness and make an effort to share your expertise with them.

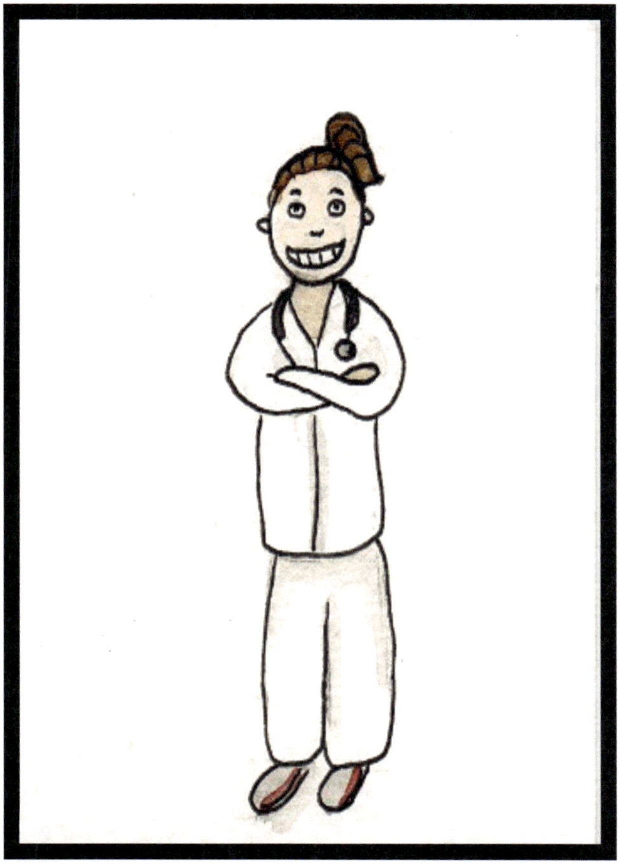

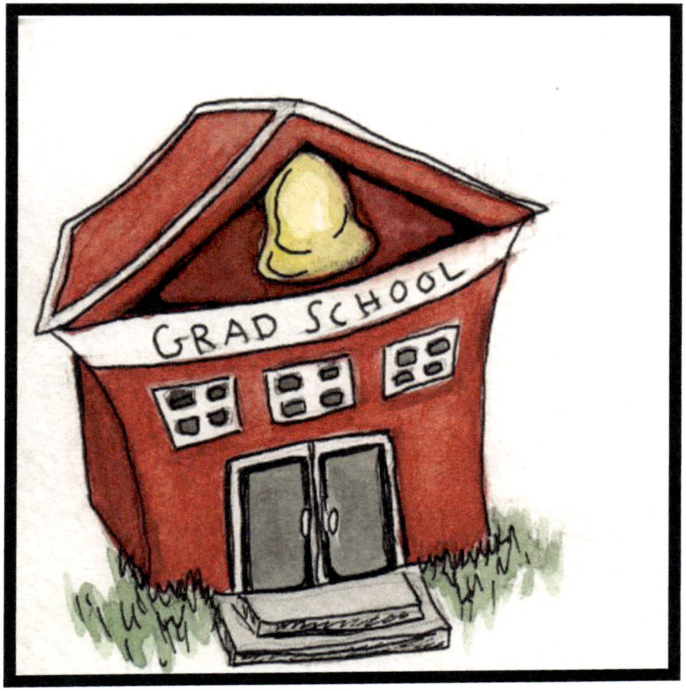


Go to graduate school in a few years; it will open doors and keep your mind turned on. Set goals, aim high and strive to reach your potential. One of the greatest perks of being a nurse is that the learning opportunities are endless. There is an amazing profession out there waiting for you. Leave your mark in a positive way. I hope you **LOVE** being a nurse.

# WELCOME TO THE PROFESSION!

Made in the USA
Monee, IL
05 November 2026

67381720R00019